World Health Organization

AFFORDABLE TECHNOLOGY

BLO[...] DEVICES [...]IGS

WHO Library Cataloguing-in-Publication Data

Affordable technology : blood pressure measuring devices for low resource settings.

1.Blood pressure determination – standards 2.Blood pressure determination – methods
3.Blood pressure determination – instrumentation 4.Diagnostic equipment – economics
5.Cardiovascular diseases – prevention and control 6.Developing countries I.World Health Organization.

ISBN 92 4 159264 8 (NLM classification: WB 280)

Printed in France

Contents

Background

Hypertension is as prevalent in many developing countries as it is in developed countries, and is an increasingly common health issue worldwide (1). It is a major risk factor for heart attacks and strokes: approximately 62% of cerebrovascular disease and 49% of ischaemic heart disease are attributable to suboptimal blood pressure (systolic blood pressure > 115 mmHg) (2). Worldwide, high blood pressure is estimated to cause 7.1 million deaths per year, with close to 4.2 million of these occurring in developing countries (2).

Blood pressure measurement in low resource settings

The treatment of hypertension has been associated with an approximate 40% reduction in the risk of stroke and 15% reduction in the risk of myocardial infarction (3). However, in developing countries the detection of major cardiovascular risk factors, such as hypertension, is often missed. Failure to identify hypertension is largely due to the unavailability of suitable blood pressure measurement devices and the limited attention paid to the techniques and procedures necessary to obtain accurate blood pressure readings (procedures for blood pressure measurement are described in Annex 1).

The treatment of hypertension has been associated with an approximate 40% reduction in the risk of stroke and 15% reduction in the risk of myocardial infarction.

There are several barriers to accurate and affordable blood pressure measurement, particularly in developing countries. These include:

- The absence of accurate, easily-obtainable, inexpensive devices for blood pressure measurement;
- The frequent marketing of non-validated blood pressure measuring devices;
- The relatively high cost of blood pressure devices given the limited resources available;
- Limited awareness of the problems associated with conventional blood pressure measurement techniques;
- A general lack of trained manpower and limited training of personnel.

To fulfil the requirements related to blood pressure measurement in low resource settings, a blood pressure measuring device should therefore be affordable and extremely simple to use, but at the same time be accurate and robust so that it can be easily used for repeated blood pressure measurements.

Meeting of experts on integrated management of cardiovascular risk, July 2002

In July 2002, WHO held a meeting to develop a package of tools for integrated cardiovascular risk assessment and management (4). The resulting *WHO CVD-Risk Management Package for Low- and Medium-Resource Settings* consists of clinical protocols for the management of cardiovascular risk, primarily in individuals detected to have hyper-

Blood pressure measuring devices for use in low resource settings should be affordable and simple to use, but at the same time be accurate and robust so that they can be easily used for repeated blood pressure measurements.

tension or diabetes through opportunistic screening (5). The availability of a reliable blood pressure measurement device was considered to be a prerequisite for implementation of the package under all levels of resource availability.

The July 2002 meeting included deliberations on blood pressure measuring devices. The experts supported the use of affordable, independently validated electronic devices in clinical practice. However, when the use of such devices is not feasible, there may be no alternative to the use of mercury and aneroid devices, which are inexpensive and easily portable. It was recommended that WHO, in collaboration with relevant professional associations and industry, should explore the development of an accurate and affordable automated blood pressure measuring device suitable for low resource settings.

Meeting of experts on accurate and affordable blood pressure measuring devices for office/clinic use in low resource settings, December 2003

A meeting of experts was convened by WHO on December 3rd, 2003 in Geneva, Switzerland, to develop technical specifications for an accurate and affordable blood pressure measuring device for office/clinic use in low resource settings. A list of meeting participants is provided in Annex 2. The objectives of the meeting were two-fold:

1. To elaborate on the preferred type of blood pressure measuring device for office/clinic use in low resource settings; and
2. To develop technical specifications for such a device.

The meeting participants discussed a variety of issues, including the future of the mercury sphygmomanometer, the importance of device accuracy and validation, and the current state-of-the-market. Based on these discussions, recommendations and technical specifications for a blood pressure measuring device for office/clinic use in low resource settings, were developed.

Overview of Blood Pressure Measurement Techniques & Devices

Blood pressure measuring techniques

The auscultatory technique

The auscultatory technique for measuring blood pressure consists of the transmission and interpretation of a signal (Korotkoff sound) from a subject via a device (mercury or aneroid sphygmomanometer) to an observer (6). This technique requires that observers be trained and assessed for accuracy and auditory acuity, and requires a good quality stethoscope. Although the auscultatory technique has remained essentially unchanged for over a century, there is now widespread acknowledgement that it can be inaccurate due to faulty application of the method (7-11). In particular, the estimation of diastolic blood pressure using the auscultatory technique is limited in accuracy. Moreover, the auscultatory approach is subject to observer error such as digit preference and observer bias (12).

The oscillometric technique

The oscillometric technique is based on the detection of variations in pressure oscillations due to arterial wall movement beneath an occluding cuff. Empirically derived algorithms are utilised, which calculate systolic and diastolic blood pressure.

The palpatory technique

The use of the simple palpatory technique for the identification of systolic blood pressure values is, at present, still under discussion.

Blood pressure measuring devices

Current options for blood pressure measuring devices include mercury sphygmomanometers, aneroid manometers, semiautomatic devices and fully automatic electronic devices.

Mercury sphygmomanometers

Historically, blood pressure measurements have been obtained through the use of mercury column sphygmomanometers which rely on the auscultatory technique. In spite of the accuracy and affordability of mercury devices, these may have a limited future due to increasing concerns about the toxicity of mercury for users and/or service personnel, and for the environment in general (13). Some countries are recommending that mercury sphygmomanometers be replaced, while others have banned the use of mercury altogether. However, to ensure that new devices conform with recommended validation protocols, the mercury sphygmomanometer will have to be retained as a gold standard in designated laboratories.

Aneroid sphygmomanometers

Aneroid devices are inexpensive and portable, and as such have been proposed as an alternative to mercury sphygmomanometers. However, the accuracy of the bellow-and-lever system through which aneroid manometers register pressure is subject to the jolts and bumps of everyday use, often leading to false readings and the consequent under- or over-estimation of blood pressure. Thus, they are less accurate than mercury sphygmomanometers. There are shock-proof aneroid sphygmomanometers available, however these are substantially more expensive. Aneroid sphygmomanometry is also limited by the problems common to the auscultatory technique, such as observer bias and terminal digit preference.

Aneroid devices require regular calibration, namely they should be checked at regular intervals (e.g. every 6 months) against an accurate mercury sphygmomanometer over the entire pressure range. This can be achieved by connecting the aneroid sphygmomanometer, via a Y-piece, to the tubing of the mercury sphygmomanometer and inflating the cuff around a bottle or cylinder. Aneroid devices can also be calibrated against a water column, where 1.6 m of water = 120 mmHg.

As mercury sphygmomanometers are removed from clinical practice there is a tendency to replace them with aneroid devices on the false assumption that, because both can be used to measure blood pressure by means of the auscultatory technique, they can be interchanged. However, as previously mentioned the accuracy of aneroid devices can be poor, as they can be knocked out of calibration easily.

Automated blood pressure measuring devices

Given the inaccuracy of the auscultatory technique irrespective of the sphygmomanometer used, there is a need to replace it with accurate automated methods of measurement. An accurate automated sphygmomanometer eliminates errors of interpretation, observer bias and terminal digit preference. Moreover, elaborate training in using the automated device is not required, although a period of instruction and an assessment of proficiency will always be necessary. Another advantage of automated devices is the ability to store readings and transmit them electronically or telephonically.

A transition toward automated blood pressure measurement is underway. However, the advent of automated devices as an alternative to the mercury manometer, although welcomed, is not without limitations (14). Automated devices are notoriously inaccurate, although more accurate devices are now appearing on the market. Users of automated devices should be aware that devices validated against International Standards can have 25% of measurements differing by more than 10 mmHg from measurements from trained observers. Thus, device validation does not guarantee reliable measurement in all patients. Another disadvantage of automated devices is that most have been designed for the self-measurement of blood pressure, and as such it cannot be assumed that they will be suitable for professional use in the office/clinic setting. In addition, oscillometric techniques cannot measure blood pressure in all situations, particularly in patients with arrhythmias such as atrial fibrillation with a rapid ventricular response, as well as in other individuals for reasons that are not always apparent.

Automated blood pressure measuring devices should only be considered as an alternative for low resource settings if validated and affordable. Currently, the feasibility of using automated devices in low resource settings may be limited by their relatively high capital and maintenance costs. Furthermore, of the more than 500 automatic blood pressure measuring devices on the market, less than 10% have been independently validated (4). Thus, there is a need to increase the supply and distribution of validated automated blood pressure measuring devices that are affordable for low resource settings. Additional important considerations in the selection of a device are durability, the need for regular servicing, and the need for a power source or frequent battery replacements. In light of the difficulties associated with frequent battery replacement, semiautomatic devices appear to be more suitable than fully automatic devices, particularly in low resource settings. Semiautomatic devices are battery powered, however they do not require frequent battery replacement as the cuff is inflated manually using a hand bulb.

Hybrid sphygmomanometers

Another alternative to the mercury sphygmomanometer is the hybrid sphygmomanometer, which combines features of both electronic and mercury devices. Hybrid devices use an electronic pressure gauge and display as a substitute for the mercury column, while blood pressure is taken in the same way as with a mercury device – using a stethoscope and listening for the Korotkoff sounds. The cuff pressure is displayed

In light of the difficulties associated with frequent battery replacement, semiautomatic blood pressure measuring devices appear to be more suitable than fully automatic devices, particularly in low resource settings.

both as a simulated mercury column using an array of LCDs, and as a digital LCD readout. The cuff is deflated in the normal way. When systolic and diastolic pressures are heard, a button next to the deflation knob on the digital device can be pressed, freezing the digital display to show measurements. This feature has the potential to eliminate terminal digit preference, a major problem with the clinical use of any auscultatory monitor. Hybrid devices allow the physician to measure blood pressure using the traditional auscultatory technique, without necessarily relying on automated readings, but without the problems associated with mercury columns. A hybrid device with LED display that has passed the International Protocol for device validation is commercially available (15). The hybrid manometer's durability, ability to withstand shock, and calibration requirements, are not yet known.

Validation of blood pressure measuring devices

Accuracy is of prime importance when selecting a blood pressure measuring device. Thus, regardless of the type of device used, standardized validation procedures are essential (10). In this regard it is important to define standards and refine specifications to be sent to industries, as well as to provide information to assist consumers in selecting reliable devices.

International protocols for blood pressure measuring device validation have been released by the Association for the Advancement of Medical Instrumentation (16), the British Hypertension Society (17), and the European Society of Hypertension Working Group on Blood Pressure Measurement (18). However, only a very small number of the blood pressure measuring devices available worldwide have been validated (19). Information on the state of the market and on devices

Automated blood pressure measuring devices should only be considered as an alternative for low resource settings if validated and affordable.

that have passed a validation test according to international protocols is available in a number of publications, including one which appeared in 2001 (19). Since then, such information is being regularly updated by dabl® Educational Trust, an independent, not for profit educational organisation (www.dableducational.com) (20), as well as by the French agency of medical devices (AFFSSAPS) (http://afssaps.sante.fr). Elsewhere, it is important that professional devices be validated according to the recognized protocols, not only in the general population, but also in specific populations such as the elderly, the obese, pregnant women and children.

Regardless of the type of blood pressure measuring device used, standardized validation procedures are essential.

Recommendations on Blood Pressure Measuring Devices for Office/Clinic Use in Low Resource Settings

1. Blood pressure measuring devices for use in low resource settings should be accurate, affordable, and easily available worldwide.

2. Given the inaccuracy of the auscultatory technique, validated and affordable electronic devices, that have the option to select manual readings, appear to be the preferred option for low resource settings.

3. In light of the toxicity of mercury, it is recommended that mercury blood pressure measuring devices be gradually phased out in favour of affordable, validated, professional electronic devices as these become available. However, in certain low resource settings it may be difficult to replace all mercury devices with automated devices within a short time frame. In addition, some mercury devices will need to be kept for calibration purposes. In these cases, special precautions should be taken in servicing mercury devices, in avoiding mercury spills, and in ensuring the safe disposal of non-functioning devices. Mercury devices should be serviced and calibrated at regular intervals. Appropriate cuff sizes should be available, and users should be trained and assessed in the performance of the auscultatory blood pressure measurement technique.

Validated and affordable electronic blood pressure measuring devices, that have the option to select manual readings, appear to be the preferred option for low resource settings.

4. In cases where aneroid devices are already being used, their continued use is appropriate provided they have been shown to be accurate not only at the time of manufacture, but also after a period of time in use. Aneroid devices should be considered only if calibrated at regular intervals (e.g. every 6 months). The need for periodic calibration, and the recommended time period between calibrations, should be clearly labelled on the device. A simple flow-chart of calibration instructions, versus a mercury or water column, should also be provided. Users should be trained and assessed in the performance of the auscultatory blood pressure measurement technique.

Aneroid devices should be considered only if calibrated at regular intervals (e.g. every 6 months).

Technical Specifications for the Development of Automated Blood Pressure Measuring Devices for Office/Clinic Use in Low Resource Settings*

The technical specifications for the development of automated blood pressure measuring devices for office/clinic use in low resource settings address the following features:
Accuracy
Transducers and power
Cuff inflation and deflation
Cuff size
Digital display
Calibration
Environmental requirements
Memory function
Performance requirements
Cost
Additional requirements

* Since these recommendations were issued a low cost semiautomatic blood pressure measuring device satisfying the above requirements has been developed and is currently undergoing validation.

1. ACCURACY

Blood pressure measuring devices should undergo validation procedures aimed at achieving both technical and clinical validation.

Technical validation should be independently obtained by institutions identified by WHO Headquarters, and should be based on international requirements, such as those defined by the European Community, in order to get a CE label.

Clinical validation should be independently obtained according to international protocols by comparison with blood pressure readings yielded by the conventional approach according to highly standardised procedures. Information on the state of the market and on devices that have passed a validation test according to such protocols is available (19, 20). Validation should be performed in the general population, as well as in specific populations.

2. TRANSDUCERS AND POWER

Measurement should ideally derive from an electronic transducer, which can function on low power.

Electronic transducers can be incorporated in semiautomatic devices, in which cuff inflation is manual and energy is provided by solar chargers to the electronic transducer itself and to a digital display only.

Power should be solar energy charged, sufficiently for the digital display and electronic transducer, and there should be an electronic indicator that the power is adequate as well as a warning system for impending power exhaustion (e.g. digital display should disappear if there is not enough power).

The use of batteries is not recommended due to difficulties in supply and maintenance. The relative cost and durability of solar power in comparison to torch batteries that are readily available, should be evaluated.

3. CUFF INFLATION AND DEFLATION MEASUREMENT TECHNIQUE

Cuff inflation should be manual to save power. The cuff deflation rate should be 2-3 mmHg/s.

Semiautomatic devices should allow the user to disable the automated mode and measure blood pressure manually using the auscultatory method. This is an important feature to allow clinicians to measure blood pressure in patients in whom oscillometric automatic blood pressure measurement is inaccurate or impossible.

4. CUFF SIZE

A range of cuff sizes, or preferably a universal cuff to suit all arm circumferences, should be provided.

5. DIGITAL DISPLAY

The digital display should be large and easily legible.

6. CALIBRATION

All blood pressure measurement devices require regular calibration. Calibration for devices subjected to intensive use should be repeated at regular intervals (e.g. every 6 months). Manufacturers should provide a simple methodology to check calibration without the need for tools or equipment.

Information should be clearly provided on the need for periodical calibration of the device, and on the recommended time period or approximate number of measurements (recorded) between calibrations.

7. ENVIRONMENTAL REQUIREMENTS

Devices should include a temperature-stabilizing system which allows for use in extreme weather conditions.

8. MEMORY FUNCTION

This function is not required.

9. PERFORMANCE REQUIREMENTS

Durability and robustness: should allow for 10-20'000 cycles

Temperature: accurate up to 50 °C

Humidity: 85%, well sealed devices

Drop test of 1 m satisfied

Vibration test satisfied

10. COST

Retail cost should be less than 20 € (euros) for validated automated/semiautomated devices.

11. ADDITIONAL REQUIREMENTS

Instructions for the use of the device, as well as information on customer service assistance, should be readily available.

Manufacturers of blood pressure measuring devices for low resource settings should be able to provide distribution outlets to developing countries.

Annex 1: Blood Pressure Measurement Procedures

The following summary of blood pressure measurement procedures is based on the European Society for Hypertension guidelines for blood pressure measurement (10).

General advice for all techniques/settings

- Explanation to subject: The first step in blood pressure measurement is an adequate explanation of the procedure in an attempt to allay fear and anxiety, especially in nervous subjects.
- Attitude of observer: Before taking the blood pressure, the observer should be in a comfortable and relaxed position. The observer should not rush the procedure otherwise the cuff may be deflated too rapidly, resulting in underestimation of systolic pressures and overestimation of diastolic pressures.
- Attitude of subject: Subjects should be encouraged to relax and should be advised that neither they nor the observer should talk for the few minutes before or during the blood pressure measurement.
- Posture of subject: Blood pressure should be measured with the subject sitting and the arm supported at heart level. Some subjects may exhibit postural hypotension, especially with certain antihypertensive drugs. When this is likely, blood pressure should be measured lying and standing.
- Choice of arm: Bilateral measurements should be made at the first consultation, and if differences greater than 20 mmHg for systolic pressure or 10 mmHg for diastolic pressure are observed for consecutive readings, the subject should be referred to a cardiovascular centre to be further evaluated in order to exclude arterial disease.

Auscultatory measurement in the office/clinic setting

- The following points should be recorded by the observer: subject position – lying, sitting or standing; subject state – anxious, relaxed; time of drug ingestion; arm – right or left; bladder size.
- The observer should ensure that the manometer is no more than three feet away so that the scale can be read easily, that the mercury column is vertical, and that the bladder dimensions are accurate. If the bladder does not completely encircle the arm, its centre must be over the brachial artery.
- The stethoscope should be placed gently over the brachial artery at the point of maximal pulsation; the cuff should then be inflated rapidly to about 30 mm Hg above the palpated systolic pressure and deflated at a rate of 2 to 3 mm Hg per pulse beat (or per second), during which the auscultatory phenomena described in Table I will be heard.

TABLE I: AUSCULTATORY SOUNDS	
Phase I	The first appearance of faint, repetitive, clear tapping sounds which gradually increase in intensity for at least two consecutive beats is the systolic blood pressure.
Phase II	A brief period may follow during which the sounds soften and acquire a swishing quality. Auscultatory gap - In some patients sounds may disappear altogether for a short time.
Phase III	The return of sharper sounds, which become crisper to regain, or even exceed the intensity of phase I sounds. The clinical significance, if any, to phases II and III has not been established.
Phase IV	The distinct abrupt muffling of sounds, which become soft and blowing in quality.
Phase V	The point at which all sounds finally disappear completely is the diastolic pressure.

- Disappearance of sounds (phase V) should be taken as diastolic pressure except when sounds persist down to zero, when muffling of sounds (phase IV) should be recorded for diastolic pressure. Measurements should be made to the nearest 2 mm Hg (blood pressure should not be rounded off to the nearest 5 or 10 mm Hg – digit preference). At least 2 measurements, taken at 1 minute intervals, should be recorded. Blood pressure should be written down as soon as it has been recorded.

Ambulatory blood pressure measurement

Ambulatory blood pressure measurement (ABPM) is increasingly being used in clinical practice (7). A detailed discussion of the advantages and disadvantages of this technique is beyond the scope of this document, in which ABPM is quoted only for general information purposes. For more information on ABPM the reader should refer to the European Society for Hypertension Guidelines for blood pressure measurement (10).

Self blood pressure measurement

As with ABPM, a detailed discussion of self blood pressure measurement (SBPM) is outside the scope of this document. Some general considerations regarding SBPM devices are provided, however it should be noted that there is a need for further research to determine the precise role of SBPM in practice.

Devices for SBPM include upper arm devices, wrist devices, and finger devices. SBPM devices that measure blood pressure at the finger are not recommended because of the inaccuracies of measurement distortion with peripheral vasoconstriction, the alteration in blood pressure the more distal the site of recording, and the effect of limb position on blood pressure. Devices that measure blood pressure at the wrist, although subject to the latter two problems, are more accurate than finger measuring devices. However, there are strong reservations about the correct use of wrist devices. Inaccurate measurements can be obtained if the wrist is not held at heart level during measurement, as well as if there is flexion and/or hyperextension of the wrist.

Electronic devices using oscillometry are becoming more popular and are replacing the auscultatory technique for SBPM. These devices require less training and are more suitable for subjects with infirmities such as arthritis and deafness. A vast array of automated devices for SBPM are being manufactured and promoted, but few have been evaluated according to the procedures considered necessary for blood pressure measuring equipment used in clinical practice.

Considering that the number of SBPM devices which have fulfilled independent validation criteria is small, the state of the market needs to be assessed regularly, with results made easily accessible to prospective purchasers. The web site devoted to blood pressure measurement –www.dableducational.com – can be consulted to determine which devices have been validated.

Factors affecting blood pressure readings

- Variability of blood pressure: Regardless of the measurement device used, blood pressure will always be a variable haemodynamic phenomenon that is influenced by many factors, including the circumstances of measurement itself, respiration, emotion, exercise, meals, tobacco, alcohol, temperature, bladder distension, and pain. Blood pressure is also influenced by age, race and diurnal variation, usually being lowest during sleep.
- White coat hypertension: White coat hypertension (WCH) is a condition in which a normotensive subject is hypertensive during repeated clinic blood pressure measurements, but pressures measured outside the medical environment by ambulatory or self measurement techniques, are normal. WHC can lead to an overestimation of initial blood pressure, as well as an underestimation of the effect of treatment (21,22).
- Special Populations: Certain groups of people merit special consideration for blood pressure measurement. These include children; the elderly, who often have isolated systolic hypertension or autonomic failure with postural hypotension; obese people in whom 'cuff hypertension' is common; subjects with arrhythmias in whom the mean of a number of measurements may have to be estimated; pregnant women in whom the disappearance of sounds (fifth phase) is the most accurate measurement of diastolic pressure except when sounds persist to zero, when the fourth phase of muffling of sounds should be used; and subjects during exercise.

Factors affecting the accuracy of blood pressure measurement

- Observer error: Observer error, which can greatly affect accuracy of measurement, can include systematic error, such as intra- and inter-observer error; terminal digit preference or rounding to a preferred digit (often zero); and observer prejudice or bias, where pressure is adjusted to suit the observer.

- Cuff and bladder: However sophisticated a blood pressure measuring device may be, if it is dependent on cuff occlusion of the arm (as are the majority of devices), it will be prone to the inaccuracy induced by miscuffing whereby a cuff contains a bladder that is either too long or too short relative to arm circumference (Table II). The British Hypertension Society and the American Heart Association recommendations for bladder dimensions are shown in Table III.

TABLE II: MISMATCHING OF BLADDER AND ARM	
Bladder too narrow or too short	Overestimation of blood pressure – 'cuff hypertension'
Undercuffing	range of error – 3.2/2.4 to 12/8 mmHg as much as 30 mmHg in obesity
Bladder too wide or too long	Underestimation of BP blood pressure
Overcuffing	range of error – 10 to 30 mmHg Undercuffing is more common than Overcuffing

TABLE III: RECOMMENDED BLADDER DIMENSIONS FOR ADULTS	
British Hypertension Society	
Standard cuff	Bladder 12 x 26 cm for the majority of adult arms
Large cuff	Bladder 12 x 40 cm for obese arms
Small cuff	Bladder 12 x 18 cm for lean adult arms and children
American Heart Association	
Small adult cuff	Bladder 10 x 24 for arm circumference 22 - 26 cm
Adult cuff Bladder	Bladder 13 x 30 for arm circumference 27 - 34 cm
Large adult cuff Bladder	Bladder 16 x 38 for arm circumference 35 - 44 cm
Adult thigh cuff Bladder	Bladder 20 x 42 for arm circumference 45 - 52 cm

Annex 2: Meeting Participants

Dr Roland Asmar (Co-Rapporteur)
L'Institut CardioVasculaire
Paris, France

Dr Stephan Mieke
Physikalisch-Technischen Bundesanstalt
Berlin, Germany

Dr Gert Van Montfrans
University of Amsterdam
Amsterdam, Netherlands

Dr Alan Murray
Freeman Hospital
Newcastle upon Tyne, United Kingdom

Dr Eoin O'Brien (Co-Chair)
Beaumont Hospital
Dublin, Ireland

Dr Gianfranco Parati (Co-Rapporteur)
Department of Clinical Medicine,
Prevention and Applied Biotechnology,
Univeristy of Milano-Bicocca, Milan;
Cardiology II, San Luca Hospital
Istituto Auxologico Italiano
Milan, Italy

Dr Gijs Steenvoorden
TNO-TPD Institute of Applied Physics
Delft, The Netherlands

WHO SECRETARIAT

Dr Dele Abegunde
Cardiovascular Diseases
Management of Noncommunicable Diseases

Dr Rafael Bengoa
Management of Noncommunicable Diseases

Dr Catherine Le Galès-Camus
Noncommunicable Diseases and Mental Health

Dr Anne Luyten
Cardiovascular Diseases
Management of Noncommunicable Diseases

Dr Shanthi Mendis (Co-Chair)
Cardiovascular Diseases
Management of Noncommunicable Diseases

Ms Joanna Nikulin
Cardiovascular Diseases
Management of Noncommunicable Diseases

Dr Bakuti Shengelia
Cardiovascular Diseases
Management of Noncommunicable Diseases

Ms Abi Sriharan
Cardiovascular Diseases
Management of Noncommunicable Diseases

Ms Carolyn Vickers
Chemical Safety
Protection of the Human Environment

REPORT WAS REVIEWED BY:

Dr Ulrich Thull
German Hypertension Society
Bremerhaven, Germany

Dr Camer Vellani
The Aga Khan University
Karachi, Pakistan

References

1. World Health Organization, International Society of Hypertension Writing Group. 2003 World Health Organization (WHO)/International Society of Hypertension (ISH) statement on the management of hypertension. J Hypertens 2003; 21:1983-1992.

2. World Health Organization. The World health report: 2002: Reducing risks, promoting healthy life. Geneva: WHO; 2002.

3. B. Collins R, Peto R, MacMahon S, Hebert P, Fiebach NH, Eberlein KA. Blood pressure, stroke, and coronary heart disease. Part 2: Short-term reductions in blood pressure: overview of randomized drug trials in their epidemiological context. Lancet 1990; 335:827-838.

4. World Health Organization. Integrated Management of Cardiovascular Risk. Report of a WHO Meeting. Geneva, 9 – 12 July 2002. Geneva: WHO; 2002.

5. World Health Organization. WHO CVD-Risk Management Package for low- and medium resource settings. Geneva: WHO; 2002.

6. Beevers G, Lip GHY, O'Brien E. ABC of hypertension. Part II. Conventional sphygmomanometry: technique of auscultatory blood pressure measurement. BMJ 2001; 322:1043–1047.

7. Parati G, de Leeuw P, Illyes M,Julius S, Kuwajima I, Mallion JM, Ohtsuka K, Imai Y and the participants in the 2001 Consensus Conference on Ambulatory Blood Pressure Monitoring. Blood pressure measurement in research. Blood Press Monit 2002; 7: 83-87.

8. O'Brien E. Ambulatory blood pressure measurement is indispensable to good clinical practice. J Hypertens 2003; 21(suppl 2):S11-S18.

9. Mancia G, Parati G, Di Rienzo M, Zanchetti A. Blood pressure variability. In: Handbook of Hypertension, Vol. 17:Pathophysiology of Hypertension. A.Zanchetti and G.Mancia eds. Elsevier Science BV 1997:117-169.

10. O'Brien E, Asmar R.,Beilin L., Imai Y., Mallion J.-M., Mancia G., Mengden T., Myers M., Padfield P., P.Palatini P., Parati G., Pickering TG., Redon J., Staessen J., Stergiou G., Verdecchia P., on behalf of the European Society of Hypertension Working Group on Blood Pressure Monitoring. European Society of Hypertension recommendations for conventional, ambulatory and home blood pressure measurement. J Hypertens 2003; 21: 821-848.

11. Parati G, Bilo G, Mancia G. Blood pressure measurement in research and in clinical practice: recent evidence. Curr Op Nephrol Hypertens 2004, in press.

12. Rose G. Standardisation of observers in blood pressure measurement. Lancet 1965; 1:673-674.

13. O'Brien E. Demise of the mercury sphygmomanometer and the dawning of a new era in blood pressure measurement. Blood Press Monit 2003; 8:19-21.

14. O'Brien E. Replacing the mercury sphygmomanometer. BMJ 2000; 320:815–816.

15. Graves JD, Tibor M, Murtagh B, Klein L, Sheps SG. The Accoson Greenlight, the first non-automated device to pass the International Protocol for blood pressure measuring devices in adults. Blood Press Monit 2004; 9:13-7.

16. Association For The Advancement Of Medical Instrumentation. American National Standard for Electronic or Automated Sphygmomanometers: ANSI/AAMI SP10 – 1993. Arlington, VA: AAMI; 1993.

17. O'Brien E, Petrie J, Littler WA, de Swiet M, Padfield PL, Altman D, et al. The British Hypertension Society Protocol for the evaluation of blood pressure measuring devices. J Hypertens 1993; 11 (suppl 2):S43–S63.

18. O'Brien E, Pickering T, Asmar R, Myers M, Parati G, Staessen J, et al., on behalf of the Working Group on Blood Pressure Monitoring of the European Society of Hypertension. International protocol for validation of blood pressure measuring devices in adults. Blood Press Monit 2002; 7:3–17.

19. O'Brien E, Waeber B, Parati G, Staessen G, Myers MG. on behalf of the European Society of Hypertension Working Group on Blood Pressure Monitoring. Blood pressure measuring devices: recommendations of the European Society of Hypertension. BMJ 2001; 322:531-536.

20. O'Brien E. A website for blood pressure measuring devices:dableducational.com. Blood Press Monit 2003; 8:177–180.

21. Mancia G, Bertinieri G, Grassi G, Parati G, Pomidossi G, Ferrari A, Gregorini L, Zanchetti A: Effects of Blood Pressure measurements by the doctor on patient's Blood Pressure and heart rate. Lancet 1983; 2:695-698.

22. Mancia G, Parati G, Pomidossi G, Grassi G, Casadei R, Zanchetti A: Alerting reaction and rise in Blood Pressure during measurements by physician and nurse. Hypertension 1987; 9:209-215.